flipped eye pub

Amittere
(to let go, to lose)

simple words, rendered sublime

Amittere

flipped eye publishing
www.flippedeye.net

First published by flipped eye publishing

Mockingbird and *Hummingbird* are included in this collection with the consent of my younger daughter who has a diagnosis of ADHD. *Love letter to my firstborn, My child buys a They/them badge* and *When your wings unfold* are included with the blessing and consent of my eldest nonbinary child.

ISBN: 978-1-905233-93-9

LOTTERY FUNDED
Supported using public funding by
ARTS COUNCIL ENGLAND

Amittere

When I choose the title for this collection I didn't know it would be prescient, that this year would be one of unimaginable loss. I dedicate this book to my late husband Sean – I will carry you always in my heart.

Amittere

Contents

Navigation .11
My child buys a They/Them badge .12
Ten minutes .14
In search of .16
Clear: An assay. .17
Dandelions .19
Complacence and water don't mix. .21
The Breach .22
Mockingbird .23
Hummingbird .24
Directions for an ex .26
Alone at the New Road Hotel .28
Approaching the New Year via Cable Street .29
Doing the big shop in Aldi .30
Like a handshake or a skipping rope .32
Treating an epidemic with one bottle of pills .34
Shamima and the lions .36
I don't want to be the one to tell you CAMHS caseloads are eighty plus and rising .39
Credo for the clinic at the girl's school .41
When your wings unfold .44
This room was not designed for doubt .49
The elephant on Holloway Road .50
In therapy .52
Joan of the estate .53
At Doxey Mermaid Pool .55
Grimhilde's eclipse .56
At fifty .57
Rival .58
Reunion .59

Lire les signes .61
Dizygotic .62
Twin .63
Extremophytes .65
Poiesis .67
Progeny .68
Oh Sylvia .69
I tell myself it is enough .71
We are not locals at The Waggon at Hale .72
Legacy .73
Alphabet for an adoption .74
"Use your voice for Good" .77
Changeling .79
Battery .81
The view from the back window of Children's Services .83
Cece .84
In the week before Christmas in the Leaving Care Team .86
Everything is laid bare .87
We are not those people .89
19th March, 2020 .90
Small things safe and not so much .91
Eighteen years in .92
New berth .93
No. 9- Humber Keel: Sheffield size, circa 1906 .94
The boatman and his keel as symbol for a long relationship .95
Abecedarian for the North Sea .96
It's not love unless it expands you both .97
Angular motion .99
Amittere .100
Love letter to my firstborn .102

Navigation

Without reference points,
distance can be hard to judge.

These are the years
we have been at sea.

Soon after they reached fourteen
my eldest turned themself

into a lighthouse.

I am here, a tender in the fog
waiting bone-cold and starless

beyond jelly mould rocks.

My child buys a They/Them badge

After *Alice in Wonderland* by Lewis Carroll.

Please allow me time to grieve
the you that slipped through slats in the fence.
The only place your given name exists
is in passwords on my phone,
scratched into your bedroom desk,
or next to marks on the door frame
to document how much you've grown.

Forgive me, I don't see boy
not yet, just the you you've always been,
somewhere in between – yes,
halfway through a door I have no key to,
a warren I cannot tumble down.
I am far too old to transmute or disappear behind a grin,
despite your insistence it can be done.

Your new pronouns
cram my mouth, get lodged behind
my tongue. I don't expect your binder
to always hold off the surgeon's knife
but forever is a stretch when you're fifteen;
this is not like a decision to tattoo
the word *regret* on your arm.

I watch your carpet get worn
with white rabbit circles,
it feels like your absolute conviction
is the hook you needed to rest
your anguish on, with only me wondering
why this one.

They are already painting the roses,
a whole court clamouring for my head
but I'll always be your Mum. I want you
to keep one more *Drink me* just in case,
I want you to leave yourself an *if*.
They don't know you, my love,
you can be anything you want.

Ten minutes

was long enough for him to tie a shoelace
around his neck
and hang it from the radiator.
When staff found him he had no pulse.
Today there is no *at least…*

Not even the inpatient unit
could keep him safe, even
on four intermittent checks an hour
ten minutes was too long.
No one could stop the flood,
push all the weight of water back,
couldn't trap it in a box, could not
could not could not keep this child
from harm. Blame will be passed around
like a parcel no one wants to be holding
when the music stops. The truth is it is
no one's fault: they all… all of them tried.

I think of mine. All the chunks of time
since I dropped you off at uni,
around 3,744 x 10 minutes:
26 days in which I don't know where you are,
who you are with. I cannot keep you here
anymore – you are not two or four or eight…
even at fifteen, ten minutes was too long.
You are fledging, I cannot catch you.

Behind my eyes are piles of Paracetamol,
Bic razors, Dettol, silence. A repurposed kitchen
knife, hoodie cord as ligature, ugly slurs.
Duracell small enough to swallow,
hand sanitizer left in the toilet,
walls like gun towers.
Isolation, a door lock
that cannot be picked from outside.

I wanted, I wanted to head to the coast,
let the wind scrape out my mind, the sea batter me
but not today. Joy Lane leads to the beach
except I find mounds of rotted seaweed
under a fish-scale sky, doubt, a rash of flies,
a jellyfish flopped on the tide
and for once I don't feel like swimming.

In search of

No one told the crocuses, or the magpies
still showing up in twos, jaunty
and strutting on the roundabouts
that there is another war, it could be
any other day if it weren't for the price of petrol
and the news, a single-track looping back to before,
only this time with an outpouring
of support but no ceasefire
for the utter lack of joy.

We are as vulnerable as statues
pecked by birds, scraped away chip by chip,
or the cliffs, because even granite is no more
invincible than we are. We tried to be walls,
to be boundaries – to contain –
but ended up as old buckets,
riddled colanders where the light leaks
through like a thousand stars.
We are out of metaphors.

So, let's take the small prizes with both hands,
the sunflower seeds, the soldier's calls
home, or your own, whatever they might be,
the string of pearls cutting
taking root on the kitchen shelf,
the cold side of the pillow,
the bergamot drift from your mug
of Earl Grey, a sudden waltz
of sun making geometric patterns
on the high street pavement,
the cathedral spire lit blue and yellow
and hold on, hold on.

Clear: An assay.

You announce yourself as threat or question,
you are top line of letters
on an eyesight test.
You eschew nuance, have no bite or layers,
you are obvious, adamant,
always right.

Intrusive as the Happy Valley strip light,
your takeout order never changes,
laid out like a dinner table,
no shyness, won't tease or flirt,
no anticipation, basic
in your Lipsy bodycon, VPL flaunted,
you have already arrived.

You shout in tabloid capitals,
have the squat *is-ness*
of a No. 15 bus,
no one gets lost in your contours
– you don't have them.
Flattened as an Ordnance Survey,
your borders have been colonised.

Your needs are as simple as a baby's;
you are gusty, you bawl, you thrive.
You are toddler primary;
you have no angle, no edge.
You don't bother with niceties
– icing sugar, ribbons, candles –

you don't drip, your desires have been stated,
you are upfront, brash.

You are St Georges on Good Friday;
stripped of flowers, the clergy all in black.
You are the bliss of a swimming pool
before anyone dives in.
You are daylight, Asda cheese sandwich, routine.
You can only be read one way,
you have one door
and it has a sign.

You absolutely won't bargain or manoeuvre,
you square up every time.
You have no hidden charges,
no after the contract's signed surprises,
you can always be traced.

Dandelions

Where else but Twitter would I find a video of jackdaws
pecking a moulting deer for fur for their nests?
Or learn that sad tears are heavier
than reflex tears and fall slower
so they are more likely to be seen?
Or here, a name I haven't heard in 25 odd years,
listing his pronouns as He. Him. Us.

That *us*. There's a reason I loved him once.

My friendships are now more tube map
than the spun complication of a spider's web
but we were dandelions then, sun-bright tufts
haloed together, connected by a stalk
until time made us wraiths of ourselves,
vulnerable to gusts. For twenty odd years

I had that one friend with whom I shared it all: jokes,
secrets, losses, food, even a bed, until she stopped
taking my calls, snuffed me out on every platform.
I won't pretend it didn't sting.
She said friendships are not contractual.
They aren't but by then I was soil
that hadn't been re-potted, stripped.

But there are other friendships, stubborn
as creeping buttercups peeking through gaps
in paving slabs, as around me
people end their calls with *love yous*
that scatter like pappus through the train into town
which takes me to The Bank of Friendship,

Blackstock Road. I hope they take cheques –

I've let too much drift. I needn't have worried,
as my mate from years past turns up in a grubby shirt,
hasn't changed – it's me who's put on the pounds,
gone grey. Like the photo he shows
me on his phone, him with some old man.
'Look closer' he says
and the stranger in the snap strays

into my ex, his eyes, that mischief, could be yesterday.

When I head home,
the streets are filaments
connecting then to now.
The wisps. How easily we disperse.

Complacence and water don't mix.

A lifeguard does not pay attention
to a scream –
silence is when he acts.

Today was the closest I've been.
I couldn't see how I would make it
back to shore.

A few teaspoons of water down the wrong way
to the lungs, it only takes two inches,
even a bucket or a toilet bowl would do.

It never mattered before
with huge florescent buoys
to mark my way back, regulation

bright coloured hat, a neon float at my waist
…but today the wind was gale force,
the current callous, indifferent

and everything changed. Like the world
these last eighteen months.
Today there were no sun-warmed pebbles

at the collar of this blue-shirt lake ironed flat,
no prosecco cheers on the lantern-lit back deck
while the moon pearls the estuary.

We talked all the time, I thought
you knew me.

The Breach

Suppose I thought I could understand her at thirteen when she was the river
all churned up and frothed, or cold and brooding… and what we needed was
a thread, a means to cross but what if the bridge was not enough, the way she
will no longer countenance touch and words are a poor substitute and
don’t   because   I am a one-sided bridge

                                                                        she refuses, her exasperation worn
like rust and holes, with side eyes and shrugs: how easily does a gate become
a wall when she pushes it shut? I am on the other side my love, my chuckle
baby, my mischief-eyed girl whose clouds never plumped with rain, who wa
always the sharp pierce of sunlight
but what   now

                                                       when crossing is forbidden and no one know
not her (and definitely not me) when lines will open again. I always thought
a bridge was a chance, a join… but why then do people choose bridges wher
they give it all up to jump.

She comes back, of course she comes back but I try too hard or not enough,
with a gridlock of words, down to one lane with no going forward or back,
impasse in her eyebrows knitted, her eyes skyward, the jut of her chin, her
head turned away.

                                                       In times of war the opposing side will always
find the most vulnerable point to attack, the breach, and it is me   still,
arms are empty
            still, flopped by my sides and what is us hangs by a frayed mid-line
through these choppy years.

I wait. I watch for the times she walks back across; I don’t care what she ask
just pray it starts with

Mum.

Mockingbird

(Traditional. A Golden Shovel after Terence Hayes)

Your gasp prompts a finger to her lips – Hush.
Ever the mimic, kingfisher shade this time, no longer little,
all grown as blue-dye blush seeps her shoulders, your baby
gone. Hugs are tolerated but far more *nopes* and *don't*
Mum, with rolled eyes, more words less say
in her life; no beak grasping yet still a
claw outstretched, please a familiar word,
she only says - Mama (s
oftly) when she wants something, all you cradled gonna
fly, no more fluffed wings piled in your lap, you can't buy
back those years, mouth tight to a thumb. You
love her still as fierce as a
swan but she is restless, a gobby mockingbird.

Hummingbird

The edges of her seeped out from the mould / the drum she marched to offbea
second child who trailed trouble in her wake /
the kid who insisted on a cape with her goggles on trips to the pool /
she was always a technicolour
busy busy child /
a flicker flash of brilliance / sparkler that even a bucket of water couldn't
extinguish/
the baby who chewed up sleep training spat it out /
all heart air brain blur /
crashing through the lounge/ leaving calling cards of crumbs /
she cannot fuel those wings except with constant snacks /
her knack for collapse /
for lost and broken things / her gym kit gifted to the 7.46 am train / 3 pairs o
specs already this year /
a dinner party's worth of crockery smashed / seven trips to A and E before th
age of six/ the way she makes me dizzy /
pacing around me in a circle whenever we have to queue / light as a penny
a bag of eyes elbows knees fringe / only her Dr Martens to tether her to the
ground /
the squirm in front of the TV / I beg her to stop stay still but she can't /

her answer to everything *wait-what* /
the endless hum of her chatter /
not afraid to square up to anyone in authority answer back interrupt /
no one wants to be on the battlefront of her tongue /
beloved fierce fearless smart /
her flight path forward backwards upside down /
we don't need answers or solutions or a cure / but she might /
her *trajectory more common in boys* /
pervasive across more than one setting / the *Often* ticks mount up
her graph plotted on the Conner's form / an Atlas range she soars over/
peaks the rest of us could never scale /
she is an iridescence on her day /
we watch her spin swirl fall more often than not /
she darts for nectar
strays but never far /
she is not a diagnosis /
she is magnificent –
and ours.

Directions for an ex

If I were to draw the way now,
when neither a map nor memory
are reliable, I'd say to

take the road from St Martin's step
just one of our many landmark break ups,
cycle a slightly wobbly path
after those Tuesday evening shifts
that ended messily in The Harp,

to Parliament Squa
Remember it's one way he

It always was.

Follow the faithful line of the Tham
that flat band of dull on the A-Z
that doesn't capture the fizz, cannot see
the gleam in your eyes or how I,
as only the young and love-blind do,
lived all week for those nights.

Cross the riv
bypass the complex k
of Vauxhall Junct

(Your particular forte)
The journey never long enough,

spent second guessing if you would
pedal on through Kennington, up Brixton Hill or
turn down my road.

Those times you did condescend to
stop off at mine,
climb two sets of stairs
to the roof terrace with its weary settee,
the breeze teasing the eucalyptus leaves,
me knowing that you'd rarely stay,
braced for the slap
of the slammed door below,
the warm kiss of tea after you'd gone,

the sun long dropped in the sky.
Your magic trick somehow, to
leave more often than you arrive.

Alone at the New Road Hotel

He is right to suspect me.
There have been rooms before,
there will be other rooms.
At the old textile factory turned hip hotel,
in Whitechapel's tatty bravado,
as the thuggish heat is sucked from the day by rain
like a pinprick eases a balloon,
relief misting the corner window.
The streets outside blade sharp and taut,
the stench of garbage skips and drunks,
with me marooned on the bed,
a small continent in itself,
puffed clouds of white sheets
muffled by pillows,
with a lover whose name is

solitude

with a lover whose name is
muffled by pillows,
puffed clouds of white sheets,
a small continent in itself,
with me marooned on the bed,
the stench of garbage skips and drunks.
The streets outside blade sharp and taut,
relief misting the corner window
like a pinprick eases a balloon,
as the thuggish heat is sucked from the day by rain.
In Whitechapel's tatty bravado,
at the old textile factory turned hip hotel,
there will be other rooms.
There have been rooms before
He is right to suspect me.

Approaching the New Year via Cable Street

There are no graces here, the Thames
is no leveller for envy or scorn.
Beyond the underpass it swipes
back and forth from wall to wall
waves slap the bankside hard

as a sheen of grime and plastic
frills the edges.

Guests spill out onto the roof terrace
for New Year's Eve fireworks at a party
where entry is £300 per head and no one questions
paying twenty quid for a double. Four floors down
out front, a woman nests in her sleeping bag,

her view a set of eight bare legs in heels,
girls in fake fur who swig M&S cans of G&T,

don't look down, and totter on
past the George Tavern and billboards
where someone has scrawled *Fuk Boris*.
By mid-afternoon the next day, the streets are full
of revellers who haven't made it home yet,

in the playground, a brown-skinned man
uses monkey bars for pull ups

while over on Insta my cousin's wife posts
a photo of a £595 fruit bowl and captions
it **WANT**. At the Prospect of Whitby,
a noose still swings. We head home past families
in a Babel shower of languages,

turn the key and open the front door
to more of the same.

Doing the big shop in Aldi

The Eastern European woman who begs
at the entrance on weekends, sees me fumble
with my wallet, hands me a trolley coin.

Here where Christmas and Easter come early without fail,
where there will always be a middle aisle
and a special offer on assuaging guilt,

there's nothing like own brand cola,
or a set of solar orbs for the patio to remind me
I don't need to be perfect to be wanted.

A mum tells her boy *stop singing or I'll put the sausages back*
but he knows she won't and anyway
singing is more necessary than his tea.

The queue splits like a bag of Ready Salted
someone ripped open for a girl with only three items
and Uri on the till winks, calls me darling

and I don't feel quite so old. I chivvy myself to pack
faster than he scans so a string of kids can
keep swinging their legs on the packing shelf.

The security guards have learnt the art
of blindness, have forgotten how to run:
I'm not chasing him down for a bunch of daffs, says one.

I return the coin to my new friend outside,
just before an older gentleman hands her
a whole roast chicken in a Bag for Life.

The drinkers sat by the exit on flattened cardboard boxes,
turn up their faces like sunflowers
anointed by the sun.

Like a handshake or a skipping rope

Where the Don converges on the Rother
and the canal, where the water came up
and stayed up and whirl-pooled apoplectic
under the bridge, and shrieked and soared,
not every meeting is straightforward.

A drunk collides with the door frame
of *The Bluecoats* at closing time, calls a black girl
exotic, croons his way down Ship Hill
clutching each lamppost; the UAF chant on days
when *Britain First* came to march: in the scum,

a Stella can, deflated 30th birthday balloon,
unaccepted proposal, Tesco trolley. Even carp
wear boots, hold their ground in the depths,
immovable as bouncers, they smirk at fisherman's
hooks and bask as six youths use a lock

for a filthy swimming pool, the towpath littered
with the casings from nicked copper wire.
A suitcase in the grass spills out clothes like a crime,
the sundown water sulks beneath the husk
of the *Guest and Chrimes* factory, which might rise

unbidden into fourteen luxury flats. The trouble
with rivers is that they need to be crossed,
a bridge must hold from both sides like a handshake
or a skipping rope neither person drops, like
settling among neighbours you don't understand,

just a ginnel between the Pakistanis, the Slovakians,
and locals of stubborn heart, definitive vowels
and flint. The pits filled in with call centres,
incomers who bought their weary selves to the school
gates, the factories, the taxis, the takeaways, the town

hall and stayed. Hauling your own self up
in a town that has nowhere to go, an Adidas trainer
flung on a telegraph wire, a street bazaar, brass band,
mela, carnival, bravado, gala, skate park and bandstand,
Mecca Bingo and *Poundland*, the flood threatening

to overspill the lock, the gap between terrace houses
like knocked out teeth, while the Hasting's clock
keeps perfect time one hundred years on,
above the water where it shrieks and soars -
where not every meeting is straightforward.

Treating an epidemic with one bottle of pills

The bucket in the corner of the photocopier room,
collects drips from exposed electric cables in the roof.

The families in the waiting room spill over too,
they don't need to be reminded they are the lucky ones.

It's like bailing out a cruise ship with an eggcup
when the industrial bilge pump fails,

or thinking we could treat a child
who broke every bone in their body with plasters.

It's like being asked to bake a cake for eight – maybe ten
people and more than a hundred show up.

We find ourselves with heads as full of patients
as a dinghy sardined with refugees,

afraid when we land, only 75% will be alive.
We are deafened by the clamour of our patient's voices,

our dreams in which we tried to catch the wobbly plates,
the suicides. What if it was your child

we told you had to wait a year? In which time
their problems would have billowed

from moderate to severe. Don't think we can't hear
the hollowed-out echo of our apologies, our hands

useless slabs. We can't work miracles, can't
bring Lazarus back, but the crowd refuse to leave.

We are an army marching on contaminated water,
blistered feet and freeze-dried food packs, still we have to battle

for the girl with arms like lined paper, the boy with no words,
the father who didn't know his kids needed him,

the mother too full of holes herself to sew up her children.
All the pills and the starving, the hair pulled out, and nails bled ragged,

the pain that can't be known that turns these kids feral,
the ones who only tell you through drawings or threats or self-
mutilation,

if we could hear them above the din, could cut ourselves
in half then half again at least 6 times, there might be a fighting chance

of reaching some
of them.

Shamima and the lions

For weeks, blood letters daubed
tidemark high on a gable wall:
Shamima is British,
until someone scrubbed off
the last two words.

Oh Shamima, maybe they would
have claimed you,
had you been softer,
more endearing

but here they are, greedy seagulls,
eyes scouring for what they can grab,
happy to demand all the fish from our seas
but turning the small boats back.

They only want a hero who knows
to keep his head down,
trained doctor to help shore up the NHS,
fly boy who can score the winning goal.

Even then it's a shaky welcome
on a tower block walkway,
the lift fragrant as a butcher's bin,
third-floor balcony hung
with a blanket sized St George's flag.

So very good at looking after their own,
reserving the right to decide who that is,
who gets to come in, who gets to stay,
not quite so fond of losers, boats, lost souls.

So here we are, where your wound won't glint
like seaglass on the surface of a beach,
ready to be found,
it must be mined gently, mud scraped away
until it reveals itself, like a hermit crab.

In a Tower Hamlets therapy room
there are young women just like you,
eyes like marbles, monotone shrugs.
It's hard to sit with a girl so numb
she seems callous, a liar at best
but trauma doesn't wear a scream
like a sign around her neck,
instead, she sits in the comfy chair next to
the soft lamp, the box of tissues on the table,
won't let me get remotely near.

Not in a refugee camp that holds
the graves of all three of your children.
At fifteen how you might have dreamed
of being one of the effortless girls,
praying no one noticed your clumpy shoes,
how constrained you felt.
Back row desk, head low, demure as a kitten,
quieter than a ghost, so your peers said.

My only crime was being dumb
but a brown girl is not allowed to be a victim,
a black lad must be able to run or kick a ball,
come if you must but come quietly, preferably not at all,
banished if you don't look penitent enough,
left to rot in desert sand.

Your Mum has baked a cake
every birthday since you've been gone,
your pyjamas neatly folded on your bed,
school blazer hung on the back of the door.
Only here in your old home are you whole,
her baby.

It doesn't matter that you've ditched your hijab,
no one sees past it now.
Under the whitewash,
the letters on the wall,
a scrawl just visible still.

I don't want to be the one to tell you CAMHS caseloads are eighty plus and rising

This door doesn't open... or
it might for some within seven days -
if on a scale of 1 to ten,
your child's risk is judged as nine or above,
otherwise let's say every five months.

Pick a card, any card:
won't eat, medical treatment
needed for self-inflicted wounds,
overdose of 10 plus Paracetamol.

Yes, we keep the keys but they are made
of candy floss, no one will tell you that
getting in is not the answer you think,
that behind this door is a House of Mirrors,
for every eighty or so of you, there is one
of us, no one has arms that wide.

One guard is a liar and the other tells the truth,
one door leads to freedom, the other
to death, you have one question,
must guess the single thing that will help
you pick,

Has she made a plan?
How frequent are his thoughts of harm?
I want to tell you I am not the liar
and this is that door

but I'm not convinced
because sometimes I cannot even remember
your face or why you are here.
Most days I am a wall
where the door is painted on,
a window too high and small to see through,

a crane game where the claw always slips
the prize, a laptop bloated with referral forms
and I cannot be the one to tell you,
I cannot keep holding my hands out
when my hands are tied,

I cannot keep saying wait, wait, wait,
wait, wait, wait wait, this is not the fairground.
I want nothing more than to let you in
but this clinic does not have
the foundations to hold you.

Credo for the clinic at the girl's school

Don't take this home
even if this shoulder bag of textbooks
is a heaviness you can't shrug off,

it will weigh on you still,
crouch panting on your stomach,
it will claw at your eyes.

When your 9am cries for her mum
who was either hibernating or gone,
says she isn't bothered

that she now has a room with an actual bed,
where no one shouts –
she misses hugs, the unpredictability.

Keep your tone neutral,
if tears threaten, stuff them back
your empathy must be muted.

Don't bring home here.
In these corridors, this tiny room,
you cannot be mum –

better to be snow fox, camouflaged.
When your 10am says she doesn't know
why she feels so low after

a year in which her half-brother watched
his dad get stabbed, a stubbed cigarette life
as the carer for her disabled mum

before she has reached fifteen, do not say
you understand. Do not make suggestions
that are plainly stupid,

there are those who recommend pinging
a rubber band instead of taking a razor
to a wrist, but this is akin to gritted teeth

in an avalanche. Resist.
Never say it will be OK, you are here
to sit with them in the tremors

and not flinch. Apparently, it is possible
to be buried in snow and still breathe.
Hold still, no one feels listened to

by a fidget. Never check your watch.
Try to focus through your 10.55's
elaborately constructed lies

It is not your job to believe her, nor judge
or call her out. Your 12.15 doesn't
come, which considering, is no surprise.

Don’t for one minute think you can
save any of them – you are sometimes
mountain ranger but not God.

At lunch, escape to the park
to inhale the sky, grab a proper latte
from the mobile van. Head back.

When your 2pm says she doesn’t feel seen,
one of ten kids, beneath a hijab she has no faith in,
tells you life is pointless, do not contradict.

When the bell goes,
leave your belays behind, do not take this home.
Do not try this at home.

When your wings unfold

"God must have an inordinate fondness for beetles."
– J.B.S Haldane, British evolutionary biologist and geneticist.

The cat has designs on the birds again
while your focus rests instead on what needs to die
to perfect your disappearing act.

With your intentions less brutal,
leaning as they do towards incision
and it's not the same of course,
when you are slap bang in front of my eyes,
the hulk of you, louder than ever,
mimicking teachers, playing Tik Toks on repeat,
very much alive.

*

Growing up, my Mum had a distant relative who was a celebrated harpsichord player. She made chilled cucumber soup when we went to visit and let us use her chalet on a beach in Somerset for holidays. The shore was insistently eroding but there was a narrow strip of marram grass and sand outside the French doors just wide enough fc deckchairs before it gave way to the shingle.

It was primitive: water in a jug, a fridge that worked intermittently, n toilet. The communal block was across the driveway, next to a woode shop on stilts that sold the inevitable seaside tat: straw hats, buckets spades, fishing nets, postcards and ice cream.

Frequently some mother would notice me in the toilets and gently or not so gently tell me the boy's toilet was next door. None of it is ther now, the erosion won in the end.

*

You haul the cat prisoner to your room,
where nothing emerges the same
as when it went in; the saggy cat exits
as a streak of speed. Inside you
keep all your soft girl edges.

The unassailable smell is not just
the trappings of grief, not quite,
just youth I think,
which will pass.

*

It seemed like there were acres of time on those holidays. When my twin and I were not being packed off to The Beach Mission, we would swing our legs on the tide wall. One time, a dad was playing football with his children and the ball came our way. When I tossed it back he shouted *thanks son*, and I liked it. I liked being mistaken for a boy but I never felt like one, tomboy suited me fine.

*

Beetles survived the K/T extinction
thought to have wiped out dinosaurs.

They are resilient, adept at adaptation.

Metamorphosis allows the young and adults
of the same species to occupy different niches
(niche as in how a living thing fits
into the world around it.)

A wasp beetle mimics its namesake
to protect itself from predators.

In Ancient Egypt, scarab beetles
symbolised rebirth, regeneration.

*

The new you shoulders out
the past, is either manic and bouncing
or gruff, sullen, rigid.
There are two of you in my mind,
I love them both.
While I clutch in my hands
the letters of your old name,
stroke each one like rosary beads,
there is no place for prayer here –
something more than resignation
not quite yet acceptance.

*

Back at home on weekends, the local kids would congregate around a rope swing on one of the mounds in the woods next to the rec. I never knew then that those mounds were Bronze Age bowl barrows, they were just small hills we didn't question.

*

On the edge of the tarmac, at playtime, the small orb I found, perfectl spherical in my palm, unfurled into a woodlouse.

*

The other kids didn't know how to take me. Sometimes they goaded me to strip to prove I was a girl. Perhaps we cared more about what's underneath than we realised. I would keep swinging or saunter off if I felt uncomfortable, but it was a nice suburban town, except for that time two older lads followed me home flicking a lighter in my face.

*

I won't call you caterpillar,
you did not eat yourself into a stupor,
to come forth triumphant and glorious;
you were not crawling or ugly,
not maggot becoming beetle,
nor snake shedding skin.

While the cavern of your room
could be chrysalis or alchemist's lair
and although you may be iridescent,
the shine of your armour braced against
the taunts on the train platform,
or the walk to school, little beetle,
you were never less before,
nor less now.

*

Perhaps you are also cat,
with two lives not nine,
the dumpy ball of fur languid in my lap,
turned sinuous hunter outside.
Are you trying out costumes, or statue?
I don't think either of us can be sure.

*

We were the kind of twins whom no one ever believed were twins. Th
relative of my mum's who wasn't related had a girlfriend in the days o
the beach chalet and she was a graphologist. When my twin and I wer
eight, she analysed our handwriting for a book she was writing.

In mine she noted *there are no signs of instability in this writing*'. In my sister's, she drew attention to the slightly rising and downward trend of the lines revealing that she was perhaps to become more moody tha
me.

*

I gather up your shed skin,
the husk from your floor,
nag you to keep some semblance of tidiness.
I will be here when your wings unfold,
not moth, cat, beetle, or gold.

This room was not designed for doubt

All three of us
know the girl he was
is absolutely not here,

he has shoved her under his bed
with his L.O.L dolls, his ice cream skirt.
This child has use only for blue,

for dirt, his trampoline, his leathered dinosaur,
is too busy flinging himself at the lino,
to allow for any talk or thought.

A climbing the furniture boy,
a clambering under the table, growling
BE QUIET at his mum kind of boy.

My children are convinced
I cannot call it work to mould play dough,
build dens, in a room where the sofa

has no more give than a bullet,
colours slabbed as alphabet blocks,
the strip light bleaching and definitive.

I take a breath, begin to dismantle
fingertip by fingertip
the certainty they came with,

see it for the snail shell
it is, offer up a blank white sheet
to draw whatever he chooses.

The elephant on Holloway Road

You would think being huge and incomparably smart
would be enough. The elephant has
no predators in the wild- except us

but it's always about power and by power I mean status, wealth, class.
The point is without them, what lengths we would go to, to survive, th
point is

how could it be an elephant
who feels grief, who uses her trunk
to entwine with another in greeting
or wraps it around her young for reassurance
and could trample someone to death?
How could all that weight and bulk
and 25mph of speed be captured and enslaved?

I sat in a meeting yesterday and heard about a boy whose house is hel
together by mess. His mother rarely leaves her bed, so, at twelve, he is
her carer. He has no one he can call for help. He smells, he cuts himse
greasy lanks of hair curtain his face and do nothing to protect him fro
being bullied, of course, while a therapist with her diamond cut vowe
her beautiful shirt, muses on how this is even possible: says, *No one is this poor, what do they live on*? As if she has never heard of benefits in
London,

where grey walls loom
like an elephant's steep back
and every day in clinic I see children
with hollow eyes who are genuinely afraid
of being stabbed,
where deprivation is a certainty

and no one is even trying to climb out,
just getting by, while the next street is
jewelled by fancy glass in front doors,
private schools and Smeg fridges
and who even knows
what the rich have in their houses?
Perhaps a piano in the corner
with ivory keys.

In therapy

Beyond the windows are hills
that look close enough to touch.
I wish I could, but I am trapped
with a child who makes a cell
of this benign space, who is about
to throw a die cast red car at my face.
I cannot use my hands as a shield.

Instead I stay poised and taut,
remember the last time: my split lip,
the shame of running through corridors
after a six year old.

In this room where the doll's house looms
in the corner, hard plastic figures
are imbued with a life of their own,
not least the decapitated man
he has jammed behind the radiator.

When I was young and adults asked:
What do you want to be when you grow up?
I was never one to say astronaut,
trapeze artist, superhero, clown.
I longed for only one job: Librarian,
friend to all those books.

Now he furiously scribbles
on his arms with green felt tip
fervently believing he is *The Hulk*,
or loops Sellotape around his fingers
shooting the ring of it out as *Spider-Man*.
We are shackled here together;
what we need is the same.

Joan of the estate

At nineteen she had licence to advise
even the king. Ordinary until she insisted
she had a hotline to God, nothing more irritating
than a girl who won't stop
going on about her thoughts.

Patron saint of the they/thems –
belligerence and fringe,
talisman of the in-betweens,
hands stuffed in the pockets
of oversized jeans,

patron saint of the ones so extreme
and rigid, they don't need
a clinic to know they're on the spectrum.
Influencer of virgin weirdos everywhere,
whose visions have them sectioned:

the girl who sees fresh bread blacken with mould,
another who hears opera when the sky unfolds,
hers came with the suffocating cloy of lilies,
when the only available labels
were heretic or witch – they couldn't let her win,

they couldn't let her live.

Joan of the precinct, Joan of the estate,
early advocate of *one life live it*,
with her supersize ideas, her penchant
for men's clothes a precaution against rape,
she was never going to be ignored,

both darling and shunned, both blessed and cursed.
Just that little bit *out there,* no one knows
what to do with a girl who insists, a girl
with zero deference, put her on a pedestal
or on a pyre

but they couldn't let her triumph,
they couldn't let her be.
How do you even argue
with God's self-appointed poster girl?
That singularity of mind, capacity to inspire,

deserves to be remembered – and nine
centuries on she's as household as Fairy,
Hoover, Marigold. Queen of all those girls
who refuse to be girls, who won't be
pigeonholed. Patron saint of the *Fuck you*s.

Of course they took her power.

At Doxey Mermaid Pool

She will not show her face; I understand.
The terrible flare of her tail, now stoppered,
bottled in this cramped tarn.
What brought her here, so far inland?

She mithers beneath the peat brown sheen,
nestled in these sinister hills and crags,
the mills and factories of a heavy, thankless past
when women were allowed so few faces,
she hid hers here, high over Blackshaw Moor,
The Roaches a crippled spine to these peaks.
She quietly seethes in her sky-touched pool,
waiting, they say, to drag in ramblers,
as duckweed drips from her horrible mouth.

No beast will drink here, no bird
fly overhead. Here where the water
is too hole-black for me to brave a swim,
closed in by clouds, a pond
where a pool has no place to be,
me and the mermaid have reached the age
of hag: why would we want to be seen?

When the world is done
with women like us, we retreat.

Grimhilde's eclipse

When no one contradicts my protests
I turn to an imperfect mirror, ask for lies.
These clicks, hearts and likes

give too many hollow replies;
frustrated, I stay here and cling.
My eldest has no need to try;

if admiration became leers I would spring
she-wolf to protect her. Have I held to her lips
a poisoned apple while doves sing?

As buds bloom on her chest would
I prune them? The cellar calls.
She is ember to my coal, I am eclipsed,

my body collapsed upon itself; a sinkhole.
She tracked my face with laughter lines
but I lack the grace, not yet ready to be invisible.

I'm castled by reflections, while my girl shines.

At fifty

Over Swalecliffe beach, clouds are rolls of fat,
sky strained blue, child in wellies, jaded sun,
gull shit on groyns. I'm unnoticeable
until I shrug off my clothes, full tilt run
for the easy reassurance of waves.
They shush me as they gentle the shoreline,
inattentive but they'll take my weight, save
me. Horizons were never meant to be mine,

could not be admired, caught and netted
like pearls and kept. Instead the ocean's hurl
exfoliates stones, once taut flesh now soft,
whatever is lost to age and life's whirl
means nothing here. The belligerent tide
will of course be back. Let it come. I tried.

Rival

Wanting to look the big man
in front of his mates, pointing
to the skiff far out on Bala's milky expanse
while I was already down to bra and pants
and wading in. The water was more comforting than bed
for a girl like me, never happier than
nuzzling into the water's neck,
each stroke reciprocating her touch,
diving into a duvet of waves
without a backward glance
in a seduction of days
when it seemed the sun never broke
through, the lake ethereal and misted.

Reunion

The Spain I remember is twenty-six years
faded, where I wore my youth carelessly
in that puritan room
in a pension in the old town
where a cello promised daily
through the central atrio, my dresses fitted
and I didn't notice what trace
I left in the world.

I do now, when I am
more often than not invisible
my baggage lumped in this suitcase,
the airport scanners not programmed
to detect menopause.

I feel twinned to this city, its central river
dammed because preservation is a necessary
response to arid months, the vivacity
giving in to moss, resignation, mud,
sweat, graffiti and a stench of drains.

Yesterday we took the train to Caminito Del Rey,
clung to wooden walkways strung 100m
above the river gorge. I have been
clinging for some time now.

I am leaving a dusting of husks,
a litter of unfinished poems,
their little skins too shrivelled to hold fruit,
their carcasses picked clean of flesh, drunk
in one flip flop at the ocean's edge.

I see myself back in a halter neck,
sauntering through the sanctity of evening cool,
looking for a taverna for cheap sangria, a meal.

I'm still here.
The sun will coax me to bud again –
for myself this time.

Lire les signes

The sun rattles her chains
over an embarrassment of views
as the world comes to the boil.

At this age my fear of risk has ratcheted up,
these thread-thin roads are wound tighter
than a retro telephone cord around
the mountain's throat. Cars squeeze past
too close to the dizzying edge.

The website suggests just a few more bends.
I always wonder which signs to trust:
lone magpie, black cat, comet.

We trudge on for the promise
of a window of glacial water, my life
choices have shrunk to reverse ripples.
Ahead the improbable turquoise
of the reservoir and a board that says:
Baignades et canotages interdits!
Risque de montées soudaine des eaux
Meme par beau temps.

I think I hear someone cry out,
it might be me.

I turn my back on the shore,
wade in.

Dizygotic

Call it genetics, call it effort
or both, that forced us away

from being mirrors to their inverse,
whole continents sometimes.

You were turtle to my porpoise,
craved the sand to bask with a book

while I would tack over the stones
into the North Sea, willing the waves

to pull me in with their delicious cold,
drag me far enough out to be alone for once.

Which doesn't mean I don't still long to retu
to you in that hard ferocious su

where geckos flicked quick as light switch
over baked clay wa

the soothe of hibiscus cooled our throa
a close night punctuated by the call to pray

Hardly out of the door already cloyed in sw
as bare-legged children chased the je

chanting mzungu; begging for minties, coins, bir
Where for the first time no one cou

tell us apart, whiteness twinning
there like it never had at hor

Twin

Not two magpies
like commas on a branch,

nor bookends where to remove one
means the whole row will collapse,

not matched as in matching
but well matched as in chess,

not two halves of an apple but joined
still to our roles.

No one could remember
whose name belonged to whom,

incomplete, together even before birth,
always *The Twins*.

Her popularity to my awkward,
her money to my lack of,

my part to protect,
see her through,

with all the wisdom of my extra
six minutes in the world.

Hers to take, expect,
forget to ask how I am.

Instead she gave in other ways;
the rings she had made

for our birthday. Both
with a moonstone orb,

daybreak ocean in a swirl
of sea fret, capture of our eyes

and of course, she asked for them to be different,
set in bands of silver, mine hammered, hers smooth.

Extremophytes

The air gets meaner as we walk up.
Inevitable, cousin, that we think of them
here, our mothers who grew in uncertain soil:
not cherished, made to feel small.

Why else would they stuff every minute
with work, *lazy* an echo they can't shrug off;
family get-togethers where we rolled eyes
as they ruthlessly vied with each other
for the best trifle crown.

We can't blame them.

The raised eyebrows, pursed lips,
endless, exacting appraisal of our weight,
each compliment threaded with fault
like blue mould veined through stilton.

We are clamped into a ski lift in July heat,
hemmed between our mothers' sighs
and our children's scorn as age settles
on us as mist wrinkles the peaks.

Beneath our feet lichen spreads its pretty lace

over rocks, Alpine Toadflax peeps out
from stone arms – the charm of tiny purple faces,
baby roots clinging fiercely to so little earth.
The supply of rain is meagre,

sun more brutal

than our mothers ever were and still they self-seed,
go on being, regardless. At the summit,
bellflowers wave – defiant little flags – for no-one.
They wait in the cracks, these small gifts,

despite odds stacked high enough to graze the clouds.

Poiesis

(for mum)

She with her fabric, needle, thread:
when I wasn't yet a maker,
she was whipping up clothes,
then tiny versions of herself,
not her exactly but close,
her body a magician's pan to conjure doves,
her womb a mixing bowl filled with dough
meter - mother - mater- matter,
raw material to create something
out of nothing – almost.

On the phone tonight I told her
of the half dead fern I bought,
how I'll try to nurse it back to life.
You're good with broken things she said
It's what you do -

both of us suckers for a project,
she could always craft something beautiful,
knew how a hole only needs a stitch,
that to mend anything is a gift.

This is what she gave me
who could only seam crooked,
was known to sew pockets on upside down
and could never fathom a pattern,
who chose pen and paper, began to sew.

Progeny

After Stillborn *by Sylvia Plath.*

These poems are magnificently alive but just not
right. They were such promising babies –
now look at them! Their silly grins,
their bug-eyed stares. See how I clapped
and cheered, pushed them onto the stage,

their pirouettes collapsing, puckered little faces
shiny with tears. No one's fault but mine,
blind and stupid with love, as most mothers are.
Not for them white socks that stay pristine;
instead, bubbled snot, chewed sleeves –

they have not found the tipping point
between brilliance and disaster. They peer
and blink behind my knees, cling to the light,
cannot fathom why they are not revered,
that they were never destined for immortality.

Oh Sylvia

Evening creeps up
too early on the afternoon,
in a midwinter nowhere near
as cold as your last
but just as dark and piercing,
like being splintered
all over from falling through glass.

I have not gone so far
as to imagine solace
could be found outside
the small sticky circle

of my child's arms, her tumbled curls,
the profound wisdom
of her head tilted pronouncements

yet I am trapped in my own hinterland
as I pad between bed and bath, fevered
and fog-headed, praying for the sun to return
and settle me like a pat on my arm.

It wasn't enough for you. a tulip stamen,
your baby's unrelenting wants became tentacles
to suck at you, ashen and suffocate your lungs.

I wish your need to escape
the drudge prison
of motherhood could
have been understood.

You are not the only one to crouch
in the breezeway under a house,
joker in the pack,
cheek pressed hard into soil,
not wanting to be found
but some of us
are digging a way out.

I tell myself it is enough

to know this road leads to the coast,
that there is no cost to looking
and although some days
Chatham's tower blocks are eyesores, today
they give the most delicious shade.

No one planted the sea thrift;
it came up anyway on the banks.
The cars on the roundabout before the M2 bridge,
are cheered on by crowds of marguerites.

When evening falls, an oyster catcher
peep peep peeps into the dusk,
it flits across the heavy counterpane
of night, thrown across the river's sheets,
with us falling asleep as the tide comes in.

Back in March, the cherry blossom was buoyant
against the rain, even the wind couldn't bruise it.
From the bus on Islington Green,
inching its way through pigeon grey streets,
a glimpse of blue and white deckchairs
on the roof above *City Hair* –

two women swigging cans of beer.
I wish my mind would settle.

We are not locals at The Waggon at Hale

An oak over the lane droops
heavy with summer,
frogs have colonised the path.

At the pub, the crowd at the bar applaud
the arrival of Ben Big Nipples
with cheers, the air white, red, and blue.

In the beer garden a man with his face
coloured in, his whole head a tattoo,
pushes a tiny girl on a swing.

We're outside too, our table by the animal
pens; the questioning snuffles of the pigs,
a bear hug of warm air.

Legacy

Parity should not be a sea that can't be grasped
but a rope held out to the drowning.

In the stranglehold of the river's knots,
bleak terrace houses straddle

Chatham's pockmarked slopes.
On a threadbare patch of grass, two small boys

kick a football and another rides
a bike with a punctured back tyre;

boys who might have held a bowl out once
and asked. A sullen dockyard sky leaches

over the High Street, its fat parade of tribute;
quaint cobbles outside Estelle's Boutique,

Little Dorrit, The Deaf Cat but its edges are damp
with sleeping bags and always the shadow of the river,

its grip as tight as Fagin's, snaking past your childhood
– its tides of too much, not enough – as your father

let his dockyard wages drip through his fingers
as fathers still do now –
or would if the docks hadn't closed in '84.

From here, the Medway is just as unforgiving
when those with nothing left   to live for,

jump.

Alphabet for an adoption

A is for after her social worker dropped her
off with strangers who she is told to call
mum and dad. **B**est behaviour
because being nice is all she has
to bargain with.

Chosen. we chose you. rescue
sticks to her tongue like her memory
of cornflakes with no milk.

Dad. she never knew hers.
with this one she has no idea
how to act. **E**nough. well meaning,
they think love will sort her out.

Forever is a coin with an unfamiliar king's head.
family is worse as the tree her social worker draws
spiders off the edges of the page. **G**ood
girls do not run out in front of cars
or drop their pants to poo outside
plate glass fronted shops.

Hope is a football they pass around
like it will detonate. **I**dentity a lucky dip
she doesn't want to put her hand in,
a **J**oke is supposed to make her laugh.

Kindness is not the password
they assumed would open her;
like love it falls short. **L**ucky. (see chosen)

so lucky to have them
when she could have ended up in care.
as continuums go, its not great.

Mum. two mums now to be exact.
will her real one come back?
Not before she turns eighteen
which feels like never.

Order helps. disney princesses lined up,
crayolas rainbowed, books by genre on her shelf.
P*lease can I go home*? she pushes them away
with a mulish will. **Q**uestions.
they say she can ask anything she wants.

Risk is complicated (c.f. safety and order)
sometimes it's what she knows;
chaos has its own calm.

Safety (1) she can't explain why she runs
away from the zone 4 house
with her own room, the meals that come
more reliably than trains. **S**iblings (2)
she has to leave this blank.

Trust. there are not enough words for this,
she replaces it with test – or is it trap?
Umbilical cord before the snip. *why*
couldn't she keep me? there is no answer
she understands.
Versions: there are many.
they do not add up, there are still gaps.

W is for wait. watch the door,
and far too many words. **X**
is the place to sign her name

if she can just remember which one.
Y. why isn't she grateful?
this is cheating which feels apt
and anyway, why not?

Z. there is no z, no neat ending
- don't ask for one.

"Use your voice for Good"

Behind the motto
at our daughters' school,
their *Black Lives Matter*

header on Instagram, protests
about a student's racist comments
on Snapchat were deleted, blocked, shut down

because pretending something
isn't there means it doesn't exist-
like a cyst say,

or electricity, or you know,
8 minutes and 46 seconds
caught on camera.

The endless news renders me inert,
all too easily indignant
about an accusation, not the thing itself

but I start to feel
like I'm wearing a t-shirt
for a band I've never heard.

Gagging isn't exactly what we chose
when we filled in the forms
for grammar school.

Emoji's, post likes and Tik Tok
won't distract my girls
from seeing we handed them a rope,

silence is like pouring water
on a chip pan fire and thank God,
they are mutinous.

Changeling

This boy is a balloon with its string cut.
Tethered doesn't mean trapped when
all
he's
ever
known
is
falling
but he came to them too late:
kind is too flimsy when the risks
rising.
and
wide
sky
are

No one could have prepared them
for how much he would scream:
a blunt object to the head
or a flood that seeps until mouths
are only just above the water line,
as intrusive as sirens when he is
too
submerged
to register

Please stop please
stop please stop please

Who really trusts the second time around
let alone the third or fourth?

                                                                  or to pop…
                                                         to the sky
                                                to be lost
                                          outcomes
                                     few
                               has

                balloon
a loose

Their job is to keep him, attach him to them
however much he tugs, hearts a bloodied mess
pulled out from their chests,
                                             hanging

Battery

She was longed for
like a Christmas present
that turned out to not be what they wanted.

They were clear on the adoption form;
no child born crack addicted
but this is who they got.

She has polarities,
with a satisfying ratio of weight to power,
her best trick always sabotage.

Communicating with her
is like shouting down a loose string
between paper cups.

In therapy she will not tolerate
questions about before,
trashes my room

when she's had enough.
Her stock phrases are
No,   *I don't care.*   *Shut up*!

Her parents can't trust her
with a phone when she doesn't see
danger; driven by quests for love.

Her place in this family a sore thumb,
she pees on her bedroom carpet,
thinks her chips are laced with bleach.

Therapeutic parenting won't stop
her running, she will chew through
the fuse of this terribly nice family,

she can't let herself be
touched by their unconditional love,
it feels too close, too hot.

They will try and try and keep
trying. As will she –
in her own thunderous way.

The view from the back window of Children's Services

In the two yards below me, each child
is placed according to the lottery
of which parents they got; the ordinary
ones who drop their kids off for childcare

in the lush square with the sandpit, trees and toys,
or the foster carers who deliver kids to a square
of bare concrete, plastic grass, awkward hugs.
This is not a game.

Sound drifts up through the grilles. We hear
the cries. All the cries.
Who in their right mind slapped a nursery
next to a contact centre?

On one side, shade; on the other, very little
grows. There is no nuance in neglect.
Nothing prepares me for being in reception
when families arrive, even when I know why,

even when I don't. There are no winners
when little ones are saying goodbye to Mum
and Dad who came arms weighed down
with Lidl bags stuffed full of promises made

too late and family packs of Quavers,
leave empty handed.
In the kitchen on the second floor
there are never any spoons,

but a succulent thrives on the windowsill.

Cece

She brings with her an apple to clutch,
after every mouthful she wobbles her tooth,
wonders if the next bite will be enough.
She tells me she is thinking of a giraffe,
the giraffe she is certain the tooth fairy will bring.

She picks up black sugar paper,
scribbles every colour
in a jungle of defiance,
proudly forms
the four letters
                of
  her
                          name,
                                  adds Mama,
                                              asks how to spell
                                   love
                 but the words
  smudge.

She knows what happens to Mamas
– this one is her fourth.

She cannot stay in this room without
calling *Mama*? every few minutes,
she knocks compulsively
on the wall to the room next door where Mama is
comes up with reasons why she must ask Mama

a question, or show Mama her picture
or find out what this animal is
that seems to have bandages on its legs
because as much as she knows about
tooth fairies and apples, she also has

an eye for the broken – how
when Mama is out of the room,
she ceases to exist.

In the week before Christmas in the Leaving Care Team

every surface is buried in chocolate, tinsel, cake. The pavements on the way into work are glass smooth. Both toilets on the first floor are out of order agai Cath really doesn't think she can deal with a crisis today. It's three degrees outside and the snow won't clear.

You cannot pour from an empty cup.

The heating hasn't been fixed for weeks. Samir admires the cobwebs on the gate illuminated by ice; aware they are still death traps. Keisha doesn't know if she's allowed to be upset. Suicide rates for 15–19-year-olds are the highest they've been for 30 years. There were 14 alleged teen murders in London this year. Aliyah isn't aware she scratches her tattoos as she talks. Jacob doesn't d emotions, only jokes but his voice has lowered a couple of notes.

When we think we have the answers, we stop thinking.

Mariella is not the only one whose caseload has increased. Risk assessment theory is no lifejacket when the water is this deep.

Even in protective clothing, the longer you're out in the rain, the more likely you are get wet.

Studies suggest thoughts of suicide are strongest for the first 15-30 minutes. Sometimes when the decision to take one's own life has been reached; the person experiences relief. What do you tell a bereaved two-year-old? Best cas scenario Paul can make a visit to each of his kids every six to eight weeks. Nobody does this for the pay. They all blame themselves. The young people on these caseloads are 70% more likely than the general population to die prematurely from unnatural causes. The last Ofsted rating for this departmer was outstanding. There are currently 160,000 vacancies in Social Care in the U.K. All these statements are true.

For the purposes of confidentiality, names have been changed.

Everything is laid bare

We keep our secrets close
but they seep out sometimes,
like sweat. Not since 1976
(when the summer was spent
in a costume on the back lawn)
did the land unburden itself as now;
a demolished stately home has wept
its ghost outline in darker patches
of grass at Clumber Park;
the eerie formal garden
resurrected at Gawthorpe Hall;
Capel Celyn under Llyn Celyn;
Plashetts village drowned by Kielder reservoir
– all become accusing, dry, knowable.
Bronze Age burial grounds appear in parks,
Anderson shelters in backyards,
although the church spire of Derwent
no longer skims the waves at Ladybower.

In weak imitation my skin becomes
a broken *Etch-a-Sketch,*
as the sun bleaches all that's hidden,
exposes tan lines, mosquito bites, flab,
the incrimination of bruises, surface
crazed as mud-larked porcelain.
Plump underground rivers
have receded to craters of dust
dark welts that twist, thirst,
fail to provide.

There is nothing in abundance
except drought. When the sun
is this indifferent I drip
as soon as I step out from the radius
of the fan. I am thrust back
to a patch of grass bitten to stubble,
when my world stretched no further
than a paddling pool
and I didn't know yet that British
summers were not meant to tell like this.

We are not those people

This summer of grass the colour of urine,
tinder stick dry, the earth creviced
as our heels, where the odds are stacked
against us like we are dogs left in cars
without the window cracked.

Our skin sticky and overripe, we are
landlocked, desperate to swim,
exhausted, mocked by sleep,
we wear our rings round our eyes,
carry inside us bricks too heavy
and painful to shit or vomit out.

Surrounded by those who wear optimism
like shades, so sure of sun they exude cool
on the underground, are still beautiful under
strip lights, who know what to say at funerals,
are not one pay day away from falling apart.

We are not those people.

Our bodies leak like new mothers
armed with cabbage leaves,
betrayed by damp stains that form
like new countries under our arms,
weighed down by dreams

like the babies we couldn't birth,
our insides are clotted with missed trains, penalty charges,
discarded lottery numbers and defiance.
We keep going when we have nothing

yet everyone still asks.

19th March, 2020

Of course, the office felt like Christmas that day.
The slight hysteria of being let out of school early,
as if someone should have brought balloons
or at least a Victoria sponge. We were giddy
with our goodbyes, confident we would be back
in no time, brandishing our Instagram reels,
a tan already flaking, Turkish Delight, nougat,
or some weird biscuits no one could get their teeth through
amassing in the kitchen and us huddled in the staff room,
pretending that seeing everyone again
was worth braving the 7.42 to Kings Cross.

But it wasn't like that.

We couldn't have known how the days would become
13 months stretched like worn knicker elastic
that eventually gave way to a baggy slack.
We didn't anticipate the mice would re-colonise,
little piles of shit like slivers of blackened fingernails
behind our computers, the coffee in the tin
a dense burial mound like the dead flies accumulating
on the windowsills. We didn't see the banners
that proliferated in the white middle class windows
shift from rainbows to Black Lives Matter,
the tumbleweed gathering on the Holloway Rd.

Small things safe and not so much

A shoot has started to unfurl
from a lemon pip on the kitchen shelf,
its tiny leaves greedy for the sun
as life goes on in the estuary,
the river spread under a big sky.

On Tuesday, a duck hatched eleven chicks
in a plant pot on our neighbour's deck,
a balled fluff rabble followed their mother
to the water's edge
for their first taste of the river.

By Sunday, none of them were left.
Duck parents are notoriously careless
with their young. We didn't know
how much it would take to wade through
the mud and meet the tide –
try to swim against it.

Eighteen years in

beneath one of those big skies –
the kind where the light diffuses
up from the horizon –
where the wide arc of the estuary
has become shrivelled,
and sludge exposed by a retreating ebb
is ugly, lined with ruts and stagnates.

On board, indoors, there's us,
sharing a sofa that has begun to sag.

It's like the way the birds I know seem
dull: I don't stop for ducks, or swans or gulls,
but the expansive shrug of a cormorant's wings,
the cut and poke of an oyster catcher's call
has me stilled, my mouth slack with awe.

What I mean to say is,
I have always loved
the waddle of ducks,
the salt-stained stench of the mud
when the tide goes out,

how I want to come home and cosy
my head on the riverbed of his chest.

New berth

Our tiny girl, safely tucked in the folds
of the canal, the field's tight swaddle,

rudely spooled into an inured sea
where she crowned the waves,

force six winds, her terror visceral,
unabated. The river mouth took her,

carried her on a contracting tide
to blink at an exhausted shore.

See how so much sky meets water
like pillow to eiderdown,

the estuary corridor preoccupied;
constant errands back and forth,

as the sun crept through the net curtains
in a cringe of light.

We left behind a bed of steel slag,
buildings with faces staved in, like fathers

whose shoulders sagged, who struggled
to smile, had lost faith in a way out.

Here seagulls learn flight on the wash,
know nothing of being tethered,

have seen the horizon stretch for miles.

No. 9- Humber Keel: Sheffield size, circa 1906

Nameless even then, born to be of use,
an old bird, never one to care about her looks.

Now I am nurse. My task to peel back
her pitted hurts, strip crumbled papery flakes

to find assailable new skin under her scabs.
Each fresh layer oozes,

with slow, tender hands I reach her naked flesh;
we have never been this intimate.

Welded together by jagged scars
and aches, I slough off her coruscation,

all one hundred and twelve years of rough.
I slather on paint like cold cream,

lay calm over her sores, bring out her gloss;
it won't be long before she shrugs it off.

The boatman and his keel as symbol for a long relationship

The boatman takes no comfort from dry land,
safety perpetually in reverse.
She is resigned, unattended on the slip,
the distance between them gapes.

Safety perpetually in reverse,
workings that failed broke, leaked or gave,
the distance between them gapes,
she's aged, her carriage as useless as laddered tights.

Workings that failed broke, leaked or gave,
when he has lived all his life for the river's gulp and slap,
she's aged, her carriage as useless as laddered tights,
there is no reward for his loyalty to the waves.

When he has lived all his life for the river's gulp and slap,
she kept out the dank a hundred years,
there is no reward for her loyalty to his ways.
The welders chalk the black; *remember how you loved me once.*

She knows it is over, left rust-coarse ashore,
The boatman takes no comfort from dry land,
his promise too thin, the message wears off in the rain,
she is resigned, unattended on the slip.

Abecedarian for the North Sea

A friend reminds me I don't do sunrises, only sunsets
But the tide won't wait.
Can it be true that all summer I have been thirsty for this,
Dismayed to find it is now too much?
Easy to be optimistic in the stillness,
Forget the risks, fire at least would take me quicker but I've been seduced,
Gaslit by his smooth talk last night, sprawled pancake flat in the harbour,
Hard to imagine being slapped down parallel to the horizon, up again,
Innocence discarded as the bow twists, rears and bucks,
Just another over-jealous narcissist,
Killers don't wear name badges, don't announce their predilections,
Look as he grins, shrugs, he is not partisan, doesn't pause,
Merely indifferent, ignores deadlines or desires, cares
Nothing for my tiny soul.
Out here, a ninety-ton keel looks little more than a bath toy,
Predictions of the weather are not facts but who am I to
Quibble when it's all I have? I stagger,
Roll, sway, everything not bolted down bangs. I feel no
Shame to say I miss the canals,
Their straight lines and certainties, familiar moods,
Unlike the nausea bubbling my throat in this Force Four to Five, occasionally Six.
Violence so close to the surface, taking the punches through my arms,
Weight strained against the galley walls, too petrified to go and pee,
'Xact locations plotted on a chart as I mutter, Please God, Please God, Please God,
Yield to my fate, hold on,
Zigzag over the rough. Pray for me.

It's not love unless it expands you both

You can always tell says the registrar
if two people should be married or not

I've crossed the undrawn line in England
beyond which strangers start to talk,
pulled in to your north, this room filled
with chatter that has the singing lilt
and fall of a nightingale
but with a touch of cartoon-
your Grandad Cyril irascible,
there was rumour that his trousers dropped
before he walked you up the aisle.

Look at you! gone full on Scouse bride,
your dandy wife to be close after
and although you've chosen to wed here,
at Hope Place, it's clear there was no need.

No one can mistake this kind of force,
like *Wile E. Coyote* with a magnet
strong enough to pull nails clean out
of a piece of wood, like a juggernaut,
that draws everyone into its wake.

The two of you separate
were already mesmerising
but together you're a garden that refuses
to be confined – everything in sight seeds:
a rose has shimmied over the fence,
a sweet pea slips the shackle of its trellis,
lobelia take over the street.

The kind of love that leaves no one behind,
as the light and noise rainbows out the door,
stretches all the way to The Mersey,
sails on out to The Irish Sea.

Angular motion

At last orders I push the door to The George Tavern on Commercial Road, instantly haloed by girls. My daughter in customised vintage nightie with lace trim, a cardi and huge stomp boots. A girl next to her, eyes panda-ed in kohl, another faery child in an enveloping smock. They are celestial, fey; I never felt so ordinary, or old.

Apparently, planets don't orbit in a perfect circle but an ellipse; an empyreal eternal loop, like I'm picking myself up from a bar after guarding one drink all night. Or that time in a dorm at Manchester YHA, waiting to taxi my eldest and their mate from a Maneskin gig when it could have been me at seventeen, missing The Cure's last encore to sprint from Wembley to catch the last train home.

The large Hadron Collider is roughly the circumference of the Circle Line. Just over sixteen miles; the distance needed to create enough energy to split atoms. Atom from the Ancient Greek *atomos*, literally indivisible but it turns out they aren't. All this time I've been in this trajectory around my kids like a superior planet, protective and encompassing. The planets go on spinning without any crank or push,

they keep rotating
as I did, as my kids do
now, all by themselves.

Amittere

At first it seemed there was no way up,
or if there was, there might be no way back.
One of those family days, so rare now,
when we found the caves at Botany Bay,
scrambled through a crumble of stone and shale,
chalk ghosting our knees
as we claimed the inside dark,
the beach and sky framed,
with us crouched in awe
of the immutability of these cliffs.

Our youngest brings all the weight
of her Geography GCSE:
It's the tension between the soluble and the denser rock,
how water gets in to make cracks, that by abrasion widen over time
and if two caves are aligned an arch might form,
which weakened by weathering can collapse under its own gravity
to create a separate column
but I can't really listen
when I long to keep you here, with me.
We walk back between the stacks,
a gap so wide we can walk four abreast

and still have space.

In a year from now,
where will we be? Salt crust under our fingernails,
a curl of seaweed in my sandal
all our eyes on the horizon again,
your applications written, exams to sit.
I'll be holding the days more tightly,
pretending not to, your passage
away from me imperceptible
since the day of your birth.

Love letter to my firstborn

Hands very definitely on hips,
stood with a bucket on your head,
or sat in nothing but a nappy
and a bead bracelet, your Michelin
belly rolls, guffaw more unavoidable
than glitter, so infectious no one could resist.

You with serious face clutching a spanner in your fist,
my heart swollen like blown bubble gum
when you told the boys at school
that a girl can wear a *Spiderman* tee-shirt
if she wants to – and you did.

The times you refused all requests
insisting it was Opposite Day
so I had to turn any yes to no,
any no to yes.

My Caenus child, with flattened chest,
bleach blond spikes, a *They/Them* badge.
My beautiful girl, a squirming wriggle
in a dress, now sharp in motorbike leathers,
called *Buddy* or *Son* in shops.

I'm ashamed it took the *Starbucks*
'Say my name' ads for me to get the fissure
in your smile, my tears all too easy
for the TV, same eyes sandpit dry
when you first explained.

You shine, you roar, you suffer and you rebuild,
you are more you now than ever,
when I park crooked saying *oops I'm not straight,*
your quick riposte. I want you to know
when I take aim, cork gun missing the line of ducks,

I'll keep trying.

Acknowledgments

With thanks to Nii Parkes for your generous spirit, your sensitivity and your ever thoughtful and meticulous editing. I am so grateful for the flipped eye family- twenty plus years not only surviving but thriving and championing brilliant voices as a small independent publisher is no mean feat and I am so proud to be part of your crew.

With thanks also to everyone who has been a part of creating these poems, either by being the inspiration, or by giving much valued feedback, or by providing the spaces in which they were written.

Thanks especially to Jack Underwood for your gentle but incisive mentoring, to the Common Ground poetry collective for being family and community and fertile soil for writing, and thanks so much to Rachel Bower for your friendship and for our poetic back and forth swapping poems for comment.

I cannot begin to express how grateful I am to all the friends and family who have held me up this past year.

To my Dad who died in December 2024 who was the first to tell me that poetry isn't about finding the best word but the only word- although I can't say I achieve this.

To Jennie McShannon – thank you always for being so present and so much a rock. To Janett Plummer – thank you for being there for the laughter and the tears. I love you both.

Thank you to Harley and Lily, my children who are no longer children. You mean everything to me and I couldn't be more proud of you both (even if neither of you will ever love poetry!) In March 2025 we lost Sean who was my love, my soulmate, and my steadfast companion through all life's challenges. He was always the fiercest critic of my writing but also my biggest cheerleader and it is so much harder to write or find meaning without him here- I am forever grateful for the 24 years we had.

To paraphrase Naomi Wood (a poet whose huge humanity is something I aspire to) we need our poems, we need to hear each other. I hope I can continue to do as much listening and reading as writing because poetry keeps me going and contains me alongside the love of the people I am so very lucky to have in my life- I hope you know who you are. .

Charlotte

Thank you for buying *Amittere*. It is Charlotte Ansell's fourth poetr collection with us. If you enjoyed it we hope you will go back an discover her earlier work. We're proud to have published Charlott for close to two decades and to have her as one of the flipped ey family. She is, without a doubt, one of our faves.

—§—

flipped eye publishing is a small publisher dedicated to publishin powerful new voices in affordable volumes. Founded in 2001 flipped eye has won awards and international recognition throug a focus on publishing fiction and poetry that is clear and true, rathe than exhibitionist.

If you would like more information about flipped eye publishing please join our mailing list online at www.flippedeye.net